How to Train a French Bulldog

Alex Parksy

How to Train a French Bulldog

ISBN:9798877066366

CONTENTS

Introduction

Welcome to "Training Your French Bulldog: A Guide from Puppy to Adult." This comprehensive guide is designed to equip you with the knowledge and tools necessary to cultivate a strong, positive relationship with your French Bulldog at every stage of their life.

Why Train Your French Bulldog

French Bulldogs are not just adorable companions; they are intelligent, spirited, and eager to please. Training your Frenchie goes beyond basic commands; it forms the foundation for a well-adjusted, happy, and cooperative canine companion. In this guide, we'll explore the myriad reasons why training is essential, from fostering clear communication to enhancing the overall well-being of your French Bulldog. Discover the joy and fulfillment that come from a harmonious bond built on trust, respect, and effective training methods.

Understanding Your French Bulldog's Behaviour

Before diving into training techniques, it's crucial to understand the unique behaviour traits of French Bulldogs. These delightful dogs have distinct personalities, quirks, and sensitivities that set them apart. By gaining insights into their behaviour, you'll be better equipped to tailor your training approach to suit their individual needs. From their playful antics to their affectionate nature, we'll unravel the intricacies of French Bulldog behaviour, laying the groundwork for a successful training journey.

Setting Realistic Expectations

Training a French Bulldog requires patience, consistency, and realistic expectations. While these dogs are quick learners, they also have their own pace and preferences. In this section, we'll explore what is achievable at different life stages, offering guidance on setting realistic goals for your Frenchie. By managing expectations, you'll create an environment conducive to positive learning experiences, ensuring a rewarding training journey for both you and your beloved French Bulldog.

Embark on this journey with an open heart and a commitment to nurturing a strong bond. Whether you're a first-time dog owner or an experienced enthusiast, this guide is your roadmap to a fulfilling and successful training experience with your French Bulldog. Together, let's create a harmonious partnership that lasts a lifetime.

1. PREPARING FOR A FRENCH BULLDOG

Choosing the Right French Bulldog Puppy

Selecting the ideal French Bulldog puppy is a crucial first step in ensuring a successful and fulfilling companionship. When choosing a puppy, consider reputable breeders who prioritize health, temperament, and ethical breeding practices. Look for signs of good health, such as clear eyes, clean ears, and a lively demeanor. Additionally, observe the puppy's behaviour to gauge its temperament – a balanced and sociable nature is typically desirable in French Bulldogs. Ensure that the breeder provides proper documentation of vaccinations, health checks, and pedigree.

Creating a Safe Home Environment

Preparing your home for a French Bulldog involves creating a safe and welcoming space. Frenchies, like all puppies, are naturally curious, so it's essential to puppy-proof your living areas. Remove potential hazards such as electrical cords, small objects that could be swallowed, and toxic plants. Designate a comfortable and secure sleeping area for your puppy, perhaps with a cozy bed or crate, to foster a sense of security. Establish clear boundaries to guide your puppy and prevent unwanted behaviours.

Consider the temperature and airflow in your home, as French Bulldogs are sensitive to extreme heat. Provide a cool and shaded area for them, especially during hot weather. Creating a safe environment also involves securing windows, balconies, and other potential escape routes to prevent accidents.

Necessary Supplies for Training

Equipping yourself with the right tools and supplies is essential for effective training. Here's a detailed list of necessary supplies for training your French Bulldog:

1. **Collar and ID Tag:** Choose a comfortable, well-fitting collar with an ID tag containing your contact information. This is a crucial safety measure, especially in case your Frenchie wanders away.

2. **Leash:** Invest in a sturdy leash of appropriate length for walks and training sessions. Opt for a leash made of durable materials that provide both strength and comfort.

3. **Crate:** A properly-sized crate serves as a safe haven for your puppy and aids in housebreaking. Make the crate cozy with soft bedding, ensuring it's a positive and secure space.

4. **Food and Water Bowls:** Select bowls that are easy to clean and appropriate for your Frenchie's size. Stainless steel or ceramic bowls are often preferred for their durability.

5. **Quality Dog Food:** Consult with your veterinarian to choose a nutritious and well-balanced dog food suitable for your French Bulldog's age, size, and health requirements.

6. **Chew Toys:** French Bulldogs, especially as puppies, have a natural inclination to chew. Provide a variety of chew toys to

satisfy this instinct and prevent them from gnawing on inappropriate items.

7. Training Treats: High-quality, small treats are excellent for positive reinforcement during training sessions. Ensure the treats are both tasty and easy for your Frenchie to consume quickly.

8. Grooming Supplies: Depending on the specific needs of your French Bulldog, gather grooming tools such as a soft brush, nail clippers, and ear cleaning solution. Regular grooming fosters a positive grooming experience.

9. Pet Insurance: Consider obtaining pet insurance to prepare for any unexpected health issues. Consult with your veterinarian to choose a plan that aligns with your Frenchie's needs.

10. Training Aids: Depending on your training approach, consider aids such as clickers or training whistles to reinforce positive behaviour.

By carefully selecting your French Bulldog, creating a secure home environment, and gathering the necessary supplies, you lay the foundation for a positive and successful journey in training your new compani

2. EARLY PUPPY TRAINING

Building a Strong Bond with Your Puppy

Establishing a strong bond with your French Bulldog puppy is fundamental to a positive and lasting relationship. Bonding not only enhances communication but also fosters trust and loyalty. Spend quality time engaging in activities that create positive associations, such as playtime, grooming, and feeding. Frequent, gentle interactions build a foundation of trust, making your Frenchie more receptive to training.

Incorporate bonding exercises like gentle petting, talking in a soothing tone, and allowing your puppy to explore their environment under supervision. Play interactive games that encourage cooperation and mutual enjoyment. Remember, patience and consistency are key; avoid overwhelming your puppy and respect their need for breaks and rest.

Basic Commands: Sit, Stay, Come

Teaching basic commands is an essential aspect of early puppy training. Start with simple commands like "sit," "stay," and "come" to establish communication and control. Here's a breakdown of each command:

1. **Sit:** Begin by holding a treat close to your Frenchie's nose and slowly moving it upward. As their head follows the treat, their bottom will naturally lower into a sitting position. Reward and praise immediately. Practice in short sessions, gradually increasing duration.

2. **Stay:** Introduce the "stay" command by having your puppy sit. Hold your hand, palm out, in front of their face and say "stay" while taking a step back. If they remain seated, reward and praise. Gradually increase the distance and duration.

3. **Come:** Encourage a positive association with the "come" command by squatting down, opening your arms, and using an enthusiastic tone. When your Frenchie approaches, reward and celebrate. Reinforce the command during play and gradually use it in various environments.

Consistency, positive reinforcement, and patience are crucial during these training sessions. Short, frequent sessions yield better results than prolonged ones, ensuring your Frenchie remains engaged and motivated.

Crate Training and Housebreaking

Crate training provides a secure space for your puppy while aiding in housebreaking. Introduce the crate gradually, making it a positive and comfortable environment. Start by placing treats and toys inside, allowing your Frenchie to explore voluntarily. Associate the crate with positive experiences, gradually closing the door for short periods, and increasing the duration over time.

Use the crate for short periods when you're unable to supervise your puppy, during meals, or when they need rest. Avoid using the crate as a form of punishment. Consistent crate training helps prevent accidents and establishes a routine for your Frenchie.

Housebreaking involves establishing a bathroom routine. Take your puppy outside after waking up, after meals, and before bedtime. Praise and reward them for eliminating outdoors. Be patient during accidents indoors, avoiding punishment and instead focusing on redirection and reinforcement of desired behaviour.

Introduction to Leash Training

Early exposure to leash training sets the foundation for enjoyable walks. Start by allowing your Frenchie to familiarize themselves with a lightweight leash and collar. Attach the leash and let them move around freely indoors. Gradually progress to short walks in a controlled environment, offering treats and praise for positive behaviour.

Teach loose leash walking by stopping when there is tension on the leash and moving forward when it slackens. Use positive reinforcement to encourage your Frenchie to walk calmly beside you. Consistent, positive experiences during leash training create a foundation for enjoyable walks and outings.

Remember, early puppy training is as much about building a positive relationship as it is about instilling basic commands. Keep sessions fun, reward-based, and tailored to your Frenchie's individual needs and temperament

3. SOCIALIZATION

Importance of Socialization

Socialization is a crucial aspect of a French Bulldog's development, shaping their behaviour and ensuring they become well-adjusted, confident, and friendly companions. Early socialization exposes your puppy to a variety of people, animals, environments, and situations, helping them learn how to navigate the world around them. The critical socialization period for puppies is generally between 3 and 14 weeks, during which they are more receptive to new experiences.

Socializing your French Bulldog helps prevent fear and aggression, common behavioural issues in poorly socialized dogs. It also lays the groundwork for positive interactions with children, adults, and other pets. A well-socialized Frenchie is more likely to be comfortable in various environments, making them adaptable and enjoyable companions.

Puppy Playdates and Classes

Facilitating puppy playdates and enrolling in puppy classes are excellent ways to expose your French Bulldog to different dogs and people in a controlled environment. Playdates with well-behaved dogs provide opportunities for social interaction and help your puppy learn appropriate play behaviours.

Puppy classes, often led by experienced trainers, offer structured socialization opportunities. They introduce basic commands, reinforce positive behaviours, and provide a supportive environment for both puppies and owners. Additionally, interacting with other puppy owners allows for the exchange of experiences and advice, creating a sense of community.

When choosing playmates or classes, prioritize those that emphasize positive reinforcement and use force-free training methods. This ensures that the socialization experiences are enjoyable and stress-free for your Frenchie.

Exposing Your Puppy to Various Environments

Variety in experiences is key to a well-socialized French Bulldog. Introduce your puppy to different environments, both indoors and outdoors, to help them feel comfortable in various settings. This exposure reduces the likelihood of anxiety or fear-related behaviours later in life.

Start with familiar places like your home and gradually progress to more stimulating environments. Parks, busy streets, and pet-friendly establishments offer opportunities for positive encounters with new people, sights, and sounds. Use treats, praise, and play to reinforce positive behaviour during these outings.

Expose your Frenchie to various surfaces, such as grass, pavement, sand, and different textures. This helps them develop confidence and adaptability, making walks and outings more enjoyable for both of you.

During socialization outings, pay attention to your puppy's body language. If they show signs of fear or discomfort, provide reassurance and allow them to explore at their own pace. Positive experiences build confidence, while negative ones can have lasting effects on their behaviour.

Incorporate socialization into your daily routine, ensuring that it remains a positive and ongoing process. Regular exposure to new people, places, and experiences contributes to a well-rounded, socially adept French Bulldog, enhancing their overall quality of life and strengthening the bond between you and your furry friend.

4. OBEDIENCE TRAINING

Advanced Commands: Lie Down, Leave It, Drop It

Building on the foundation of basic commands, introducing advanced commands enhances your French Bulldog's obedience and strengthens the communication between you and your furry companion.

1. Lie Down: Teach your Frenchie to lie down on command by starting from a sitting position. Hold a treat close to their nose and lower it to the ground while saying "lie down." As they follow the treat, reward and praise when they achieve the lying position. Practice regularly, gradually phasing out the treat but continuing to reinforce the behaviour.

2. Leave It: The "leave it" command is invaluable for preventing your Frenchie from picking up or engaging with unwanted items. Start with a treat in your closed hand and say "leave it." When they refrain from trying to grab the treat, reward and praise. Gradually increase the difficulty by using more tempting items and extending the duration before rewarding.

3. Drop It: Teaching your French Bulldog to drop items from their mouth is essential for safety. Begin by offering a toy and saying "drop it" as you present a treat. When they release the item, reward and praise. Extend this command to other objects, reinforcing the behaviour consistently.

Positive Reinforcement Techniques

Positive reinforcement is a powerful and humane training method that involves rewarding desired behaviours to encourage their repetition. For French Bulldogs, who respond well to positive interactions, this approach fosters a strong bond and a willingness to learn. Here are key positive reinforcement techniques:

1. Treats and Praise: Use small, tasty treats as immediate rewards for correct behaviour. Combine treats with verbal praise, ensuring a positive association with the desired action.

2. Play and Affection: Incorporate playtime and affectionate gestures into your training sessions. French Bulldogs often respond enthusiastically to play as a reward, whether it's with a favorite toy or interactive games.

3. Timing is Key: Timely reinforcement is crucial for effective positive reinforcement. Reward your Frenchie immediately after they exhibit the desired behaviour to create a clear connection between the action and the reward.

4. Consistency: Consistency is key in positive reinforcement. Reinforce good behaviour consistently while ignoring or redirecting unwanted behaviour. This clarity helps your Frenchie understand expectations.

5. Variable Rewards: Introduce variable rewards to maintain motivation. While treats are excellent, vary the types of rewards to keep your Frenchie engaged. Sometimes, offer a favorite toy or extra playtime as a reward.

Clicker Training for French Bulldogs

Clicker training is a popular and effective method that pairs a distinct sound (the click) with positive reinforcement. This technique provides clear communication and precise feedback to your Frenchie, making it a valuable tool for obedience training.

1. Association: Introduce the clicker by associating the sound with immediate rewards. Click, then treat. Repeat this process until your Frenchie understands that the click signifies a reward.

2. Timing: Clicker training relies on precise timing. Click the moment your Frenchie performs the desired behaviour, followed by a treat. This immediacy helps them connect the click with the specific action.

3. Consistency: Consistency is crucial in clicker training. Use the clicker consistently for desired behaviours, ensuring a clear understanding for your Frenchie. Avoid using the clicker for punishment.

4. Gradual Complexity: Start with simple commands and gradually introduce more complex behaviours. Clicker training allows for a gradual progression of skills, making it suitable for both basic and advanced obedience training.

By incorporating advanced commands and positive reinforcement techniques, along with the precision of clicker training, you'll not only enhance your French Bulldog's obedience but also deepen the bond between you and your intelligent and responsive companion.

5. LEASH MANNERS AND WALKING ETIQUETTE

Loose Leash Walking

Teaching your French Bulldog loose leash walking is essential for enjoyable and stress-free walks. Mastering this skill not only enhances the walking experience for both you and your Frenchie but also promotes safety and better leash manners.

1. **Start Indoors:** Begin training indoors or in a quiet, familiar outdoor space. Attach the leash and let your Frenchie explore while keeping the leash loose. Reward them for staying close and not pulling.

2. **Positive Reinforcement:** Use positive reinforcement techniques during walks. Reward your Frenchie with treats and praise when they walk calmly beside you with a loose leash. Consistency is key; reinforce good behaviour consistently to build a positive association.

3. **Change Directions:** To discourage pulling, change directions when your Frenchie starts to pull on the leash. This helps them understand that pulling doesn't lead to where they want to go. Be patient and reward them when they walk without pulling.

4. Short Leash Sessions: Keep initial leash training sessions short to maintain your Frenchie's attention and enthusiasm. Gradually increase the duration of walks as they become more comfortable with loose leash walking.

Dealing with Pulling Behaviour

Addressing pulling behaviour is a common challenge during leash training. Implement these strategies to curb pulling and instill good leash manners:

1. Stop and Stand Still: When your Frenchie starts pulling, stop walking and stand still. This interrupts the forward movement and teaches them that pulling results in a lack of progress. Once they relax the tension on the leash, resume walking.

2. Use Positive Reinforcement: Reward your Frenchie when they walk without pulling. Reinforce the behaviour you want by praising and treating them when the leash is loose. This positive reinforcement encourages them to walk politely on the leash.

3. Consistent Training: Consistency is crucial in addressing pulling behaviour. Enforce the same rules consistently, and avoid giving in to pulling. Over time, your Frenchie will learn that walking nicely on the leash is the key to moving forward.

4. Consider a No-Pull Harness: If your Frenchie continues to pull, consider using a no-pull harness. These harnesses discourage pulling by redirecting your dog's attention without causing discomfort. Always ensure the harness fits properly and doesn't restrict movement.

Introducing Collars and Harnesses

Choosing the right collar or harness is an important step in leash training. Here's a guide to introducing and using collars and harnesses effectively:

1. **Collars:** Start by introducing a lightweight collar to your Frenchie. Allow them to become accustomed to wearing it indoors before attaching a leash. Use positive reinforcement to create a positive association with the collar.

2. **Harnesses:** Harnesses distribute pressure more evenly across your Frenchie's body, reducing the risk of neck strain. Introduce the harness gradually, letting them wear it without the leash first. Again, use positive reinforcement to associate the harness with positive experiences.

3. **Choosing the Right Fit:** Ensure that both the collar and harness fit snugly but not too tight. You should be able to fit two fingers comfortably between the collar or harness and your Frenchie's neck or body. Regularly check the fit as your puppy grows.

4. **Leash Attachment:** Choose a collar or harness with a front or back leash attachment, depending on your training needs. Front attachments are effective for discouraging pulling, while back attachments provide more control.

By focusing on loose leash walking, addressing pulling behaviour with positive reinforcement, and introducing collars and harnesses gradually, you'll create a positive walking experience for both you and your French Bulldog, fostering good leash manners and walking etiquette.

6. ADDRESSING BEHAVIOURAL ISSUES

Common Behavioural Problems in French Bulldogs

Understanding and addressing common behavioural problems in French Bulldogs is crucial for a harmonious relationship. Recognizing early signs and employing effective strategies can prevent these issues from escalating. Here are some common behavioural problems:

1. **Excessive Barking:** French Bulldogs are known for being vocal, but excessive barking can become a problem. Identify the triggers for barking, such as boredom, fear, or excitement, and address them accordingly.

2. **Destructive Chewing:** Chewing is a natural behaviour, but if your Frenchie engages in destructive chewing, it may indicate boredom or anxiety. Provide appropriate chew toys, supervise chewing activities, and redirect their focus when needed.

3. **Jumping Up:** Jumping up on people is a common behaviour, especially in enthusiastic French Bulldogs. Teach them alternative greetings and use positive reinforcement to reward calm behaviour.

4. **Digging:** Some Frenchies have a tendency to dig, often out of instinct or boredom. Provide a designated digging area, filled with soft soil or sand, and redirect their digging tendencies to that space.

5. **Fearfulness:** French Bulldogs can be sensitive, and fearfulness may manifest in various situations. Gradual exposure, positive reinforcement, and creating positive associations can help alleviate fear-related behaviours.

Separation Anxiety

Separation anxiety is a common issue in French Bulldogs and can lead to destructive behaviours, excessive barking, and distress when left alone. Addressing separation anxiety involves a gradual process of desensitization and creating a positive association with your absence:

1. **Gradual Departures:** Practice short departures and arrivals to help your Frenchie become accustomed to your coming and going. Avoid making departures overly emotional.

2. **Create Positive Associations:** Associate your departures with positive experiences, such as leaving treats or toys that they enjoy. This helps your Frenchie associate your absence with positive things.

3. **Calm Exits and Entries:** Maintain a calm demeanor when leaving and returning home. Avoid creating a big fuss, as this can heighten anxiety. Instead, reward calm behaviour upon your return.

4. Provide Entertainment: Leave interactive toys or puzzle feeders to keep your Frenchie occupied in your absence. This can distract them from the anxiety of being alone.

5. Consult a Professional: If separation anxiety persists, consider seeking guidance from a professional dog trainer or behaviourist. They can provide tailored strategies to address your Frenchie's specific needs.

Aggression and Barking

Addressing aggression and excessive barking involves understanding the root causes and implementing targeted training techniques:

1. Identify Triggers: Identify the triggers that lead to aggression or barking. This could include fear, territorial behaviour, or frustration. Understanding the triggers is essential for effective intervention.

2. Positive Reinforcement: Use positive reinforcement to encourage calm behaviour. Reward your Frenchie when they exhibit appropriate reactions to situations that would typically trigger aggression or barking.

3. Counter-Conditioning: Gradually expose your Frenchie to the triggers in a controlled and positive way. This process, known as counter-conditioning, helps them associate the triggers with positive outcomes.

4. Professional Help: Aggressive behaviour may require professional intervention. Consult with a qualified dog trainer or behaviourist who can assess the situation and provide a tailored training plan.

5. Regular Exercise: Ensure your Frenchie receives adequate physical and mental exercise. A tired dog is less likely to exhibit aggressive behaviour or excessive barking.

Addressing behavioural issues requires patience, consistency, and a deep understanding of your French Bulldog's individual needs. Tailor your approach to their specific behaviours and seek professional guidance if needed to create a happy and well-behaved companion.

7. HEALTH AND GROOMING

Regular Vet Checkups

Regular veterinary checkups are essential for maintaining your French Bulldog's overall health and catching any potential issues early. Here's a guide to incorporating vet checkups into your Frenchie's care routine:

1. Frequency: Schedule regular checkups at least once a year for adult French Bulldogs. Puppies may require more frequent visits to ensure they receive necessary vaccinations and preventive care.

2. Vaccinations and Preventive Care: Follow your veterinarian's recommended vaccination schedule to protect your Frenchie from common diseases. Discuss preventive measures for parasites, heartworm, and other health concerns based on your dog's lifestyle and environment.

3. Dental Care: Dental health is crucial for overall well-being. Discuss dental care practices with your vet and inquire about professional cleanings if necessary. Implement a dental care routine at home, such as regular brushing.

4. Senior Care: As your Frenchie ages, consider more frequent vet checkups to monitor for age-related issues. Discuss changes in diet, exercise, and preventive care tailored to your senior dog's needs.

5. Emergency Care: Familiarize yourself with emergency veterinary services in your area. Knowing where to go in case of an emergency can be crucial for prompt and effective care.

Grooming Tips for French Bulldogs

French Bulldogs have a short, smooth coat that requires regular grooming to maintain skin health and minimize shedding. Here are grooming tips for keeping your Frenchie looking and feeling their best:

1. Brushing: Brush your Frenchie's coat regularly to remove loose hair and distribute natural oils. Use a soft brush or grooming glove to prevent skin irritation. Regular brushing also helps reduce shedding.

2. Bathing: Bathe your French Bulldog as needed, typically every 2-3 months or when they get dirty. Use a mild dog shampoo to avoid skin irritation. Be thorough but gentle, paying attention to folds and wrinkles.

3. Wrinkle Care: Frenchies have adorable facial wrinkles, but these areas require special attention. Keep the wrinkles clean and dry to prevent skin infections. Use a damp cloth or mild wipes to gently clean between the wrinkles.

4. Ear Cleaning: French Bulldogs are prone to ear infections due to their floppy ears. Clean their ears regularly using a vet-approved ear cleaner and cotton balls. Be gentle and avoid inserting anything deep into the ear canal.

5. Nail Trimming: Trim your Frenchie's nails regularly to prevent discomfort and potential injury. Use dog nail clippers and be cautious not to cut into the quick. If you're unsure, consult your vet or a professional groomer for guidance.

Nail Trimming and Ear Cleaning

1. Nail Trimming:
   - *Tools:* Use quality dog nail clippers or a nail grinder. Have styptic powder on hand in case of accidental bleeding.
   - *Frequency:* Trim your Frenchie's nails every 2-4 weeks, depending on their activity level. Regular walks on pavement may naturally wear down nails.

2. Ear Cleaning:
   - *Supplies:* Use a vet-approved ear cleaning solution, cotton balls, or gauze pads.
   - *Procedure:* Gently lift your Frenchie's ear and apply the cleaning solution, then massage the base of the ear to distribute the solution. Wipe away any debris with a cotton ball or gauze.

3. Skin and Coat Care:
   - *Regular Brushing:* Brush your Frenchie's coat at least once a week to remove loose hair and prevent matting.

- *Bathing:* Bathe your Frenchie every 2-3 months or as needed. Use a mild dog shampoo and ensure thorough drying, especially in skin folds.

4. Dental Care:

- *Toothbrushing:* Introduce toothbrushing early to maintain good oral health. Use a dog-friendly toothbrush and toothpaste, and brush your Frenchie's teeth regularly.

Remember, grooming is not just about aesthetics; it plays a crucial role in your French Bulldog's overall health and well-being. Regular care and attention to grooming needs help prevent skin issues, maintain oral health, and keep your Frenchie comfortable and happy.

8. FEEDING AND NUTRITION

Choosing the Right Dog Food

Selecting the right dog food is paramount to ensuring your French Bulldog's health and well-being. Here's a comprehensive guide to help you make informed choices:

1. **Consider Age and Life Stage:** French Bulldogs have different nutritional needs at various life stages. Choose a dog food that is appropriate for your Frenchie's age – whether they are a puppy, adult, or senior.

2. **Check Ingredient Quality:** Look for dog foods with high-quality, named animal proteins as the primary ingredients. Avoid fillers like corn, soy, or artificial additives. A balanced and nutritious diet supports overall health and vitality.

3. **Consider Breed-Specific Formulas:** Some dog food brands offer breed-specific formulas, taking into account the unique needs of French Bulldogs. These formulations may address specific health concerns and contribute to optimal development.

4. **Protein Content:** French Bulldogs benefit from a moderate to high protein content in their diet. Aim for a food that contains protein from quality sources like meat, fish, or eggs.

5. **Healthy Fats:** Healthy fats, such as omega-3 and omega-6 fatty acids, support skin health and a shiny coat. Look for dog foods that include sources of healthy fats like fish oil or flaxseed.

6. **Grain-Free or Grain-Inclusive:** While some dogs do well on grain-free diets, others thrive with grain-inclusive options. Consider your Frenchie's individual needs and consult with your veterinarian if you have concerns about grain sensitivity.

7. **Avoid Artificial Additives:** Choose dog foods that are free from artificial colours, flavours, and preservatives. Natural ingredients contribute to a healthier diet for your French Bulldog.

8. **Consult Your Veterinarian:** Always consult with your veterinarian before making significant changes to your Frenchie's diet. They can provide guidance based on your dog's specific health requirements.

Creating a Feeding Schedule

Establishing a consistent feeding schedule is vital for maintaining your French Bulldog's health and preventing overfeeding. Follow these guidelines to create an effective feeding routine:

1. Determine Portion Sizes: Consult with your veterinarian to determine the appropriate portion sizes for your Frenchie based on factors like age, weight, activity level, and health status.

2. Divide Daily Intake: Divide your Frenchie's daily food intake into two or three meals. Smaller, more frequent meals help prevent digestive issues and support stable energy levels.

3. Set Regular Meal Times: Establish a routine by feeding your Frenchie at the same times each day. Consistency in meal times helps regulate your dog's digestion and can contribute to better behaviour.

4. Avoid Free Feeding: While free-feeding (leaving food out all day) may work for some dogs, it can lead to overeating in others. Controlled portions at set meal times help you monitor your Frenchie's food intake.

5. Monitor Body Condition: Regularly assess your Frenchie's body condition and adjust portion sizes accordingly. A healthy weight contributes to overall well-being and reduces the risk of obesity-related health issues.

Addressing Food Allergies and Sensitivities

Food allergies and sensitivities can manifest in various ways, including digestive upset, skin issues, and ear infections. Take the following steps to address and manage potential food allergies or sensitivities:

1. **Identify Symptoms:** Watch for signs of food allergies, such as itching, redness, ear infections, gastrointestinal upset, or changes in stool quality. Keep a detailed record of your Frenchie's symptoms.

2. **Switch to Limited Ingredient Diet:** If you suspect food allergies, consider switching to a limited ingredient diet with a novel protein source (one your Frenchie hasn't eaten before) and limited additional ingredients.

3. **Consult with Your Vet:** If symptoms persist, consult with your veterinarian. They may recommend an elimination diet or allergy testing to pinpoint the specific allergen.

4. **Gradual Food Introductions:** When introducing new foods, do so gradually. This helps you identify any adverse reactions and gives your Frenchie's digestive system time to adjust.

5. **Consider Hypoallergenic Formulas:** In severe cases, your vet may recommend hypoallergenic dog food formulated to minimize the risk of triggering allergies. These foods often use hydrolysed proteins or novel protein sources.

6. **Read Labels Carefully:** Be diligent about reading food labels to identify potential allergens. Avoid foods with common allergens like chicken, beef, wheat, and dairy if they seem to be causing issues.

Remember, addressing your French Bulldog's specific nutritional needs requires observation, consultation with your veterinarian, and sometimes a bit of trial and error. Creating a well-balanced diet and feeding schedule tailored to your Frenchie's individual requirements is key to supporting their overall health and longevity.

9. EXERCISE AND MENTAL STIMULATION

Appropriate Exercise for French Bulldogs

Providing appropriate exercise is crucial for keeping your French Bulldog physically and mentally healthy. While Frenchies are not overly energetic, they still benefit from regular exercise tailored to their needs:

1. **Short, Regular Walks:** French Bulldogs have a moderate exercise requirement. Short walks multiple times a day are ideal to meet their needs without overexertion. Aim for at least 20-30 minutes of daily walking.

2. **Playtime at Home:** Engage in indoor playtime with your Frenchie. Use toys like soft balls, plush toys, or interactive toys that encourage movement without causing strain on their joints.

3. **Interactive Games:** Incorporate mentally stimulating games during exercise. Hide treats around the house for them to find, play hide-and-seek, or use puzzle toys that dispense treats as rewards.

4. Consideration for Weather: Be mindful of extreme weather conditions, especially heat. French Bulldogs are sensitive to heat, so schedule walks during cooler parts of the day and provide shade and water during outdoor activities.

5. Swimming: If your Frenchie enjoys water, consider introducing them to shallow pools or safe water sources. Swimming is a low-impact exercise that is easy on their joints.

Interactive Toys and Games

Interactive toys and games play a crucial role in keeping French Bulldogs mentally stimulated and preventing boredom. Here are some options:

1. Puzzle Feeders: Use puzzle feeders or treat-dispensing toys to engage your Frenchie's mind during mealtime. These toys require them to work for their food, providing mental stimulation.

2. Interactive Plush Toys: Choose plush toys with hidden squeakers or crinkles. These toys appeal to their natural instincts and keep them entertained.

3. Chew Toys: Provide a variety of chew toys to satisfy their natural chewing instincts. Ensure the toys are safe and durable to withstand their strong jaws.

4. Tug-of-War: Play a gentle game of tug-of-war with appropriate toys. This interactive game not only provides physical exercise but also strengthens the bond between you and your Frenchie.

5. Fetch: Play fetch indoors or in a secure, fenced area. Use soft toys to prevent injury and ensure a safe environment for this classic game.

Preventing Boredom and Destructive Behaviour

Preventing boredom is essential to curb destructive behaviours and maintain a happy, well-behaved Frenchie:

1. Rotate Toys: Keep a rotation of toys to prevent your Frenchie from getting bored with the same items. Introduce new toys periodically to pique their interest.

2. Create a Stimulating Environment: Provide a stimulating environment with a variety of textures, sounds, and smells. Incorporate safe items like interactive rugs or soft climbing structures.

3. Training Sessions: Engage in short training sessions to stimulate your Frenchie's mind. Teach them new tricks or reinforce existing commands. Positive reinforcement makes these sessions enjoyable for both of you.

4. Interactive Playtime: Spend quality time engaging in interactive play. This not only provides physical exercise but also strengthens the bond between you and your Frenchie.

5. Use Food Dispensing Toys: Incorporate food-dispensing toys or frozen stuffed Kongs to keep them entertained. This encourages problem-solving and provides a rewarding challenge.

By incorporating appropriate exercise, interactive toys, and mental stimulation into your Frenchie's daily routine, you not only address their physical needs but also nurture their cognitive well-being. A mentally stimulated and engaged French Bulldog is more likely to exhibit positive behaviours and less prone to boredom-related issues.

10. AGEING GRACEFULLY

Adjusting Training for Adult French Bulldogs

As your French Bulldog transitions into adulthood, their training needs may evolve. Consider these adjustments to ensure ongoing positive development:

1. **Refine Existing Commands:** Reinforce and fine-tune basic commands such as sit, stay, and come. Adult Frenchies benefit from consistent reinforcement to maintain good behaviour.

2. **Introduce Advanced Commands:** Expand your Frenchie's training repertoire by introducing new commands or refining existing ones. This mental stimulation is crucial for keeping their minds active and engaged.

3. **Maintain Regular Exercise:** While the energy levels of adult French Bulldogs may stabilize, regular exercise remains essential for physical health. Adjust the intensity and duration of walks to suit their individual needs.

4. **Address Behavioural Changes:** Monitor for any behavioural changes and address them promptly. Adult dogs may experience shifts in temperament or reactions to stimuli,

and understanding these changes is crucial for effective training.

5. **Mindful Socialization:** Continue to expose your adult Frenchie to various social situations, ensuring they remain well-adjusted and comfortable in different environments.

Senior Dog Care Tips

As your French Bulldog enters their senior years, their care requirements may change. Consider the following tips to ensure their well-being:

1. **Regular Vet Checkups:** Increase the frequency of veterinary checkups to address age-related health concerns. Regular monitoring can help catch and manage potential issues early.

2. **Adjust Diet:** Consult with your veterinarian to adjust your senior Frenchie's diet based on their changing nutritional needs. Senior dog foods often contain supplements that support joint health and other aging-related concerns.

3. **Moderate Exercise:** Adjust the intensity and duration of exercise to suit your senior Frenchie's comfort level. Short, gentle walks can help maintain mobility without causing strain.

4. **Joint Health Support:** Consider joint supplements or foods rich in glucosamine and omega-3 fatty acids to support joint health. These can be beneficial in managing age-related arthritis or stiffness.

5. **Dental Care:** Continue regular dental care, including tooth brushing and professional cleanings if recommended by your veterinarian. Dental health is crucial for overall well-being.

Dealing with Common Health Issues

Senior French Bulldogs may be prone to certain health issues. Be vigilant and seek veterinary attention for the following common concerns:

1. **Arthritis:** Monitor for signs of arthritis, such as stiffness, limping, or difficulty getting up. Provide comfortable bedding and consider joint supplements to alleviate symptoms.

2. **Dental Problems:** Senior dogs may be more susceptible to dental issues. Maintain regular dental care to prevent periodontal disease and ensure overall health.

3. **Cognitive Dysfunction:** Some aging French Bulldogs may experience cognitive dysfunction, leading to changes in behaviour. Create a comforting environment and consult your vet for strategies to manage cognitive decline.

4. **Vision and Hearing Loss:** Seniors may experience gradual loss of vision or hearing. Ensure their environment is safe and provide cues through touch or visual signals during training.

5. **Weight Management:** Senior dogs are prone to weight gain, which can exacerbate existing health issues. Monitor their weight and adjust their diet and exercise accordingly.

By adapting your training approach, providing specialized care for senior needs, and addressing common health issues, you can help your French Bulldog age gracefully and enjoy a comfortable and fulfilling life in their later years. Regular veterinary checkups and attentive care are key to ensuring their well-being as they enter the senior stage of life.

Conclusion

Celebrating Your French Bulldog's Progress

As you conclude your journey of training and caring for your French Bulldog, take a moment to reflect on the remarkable progress both you and your furry companion have made. Celebrate the milestones, no matter how small, and acknowledge the unique bond that has blossomed between you. Whether it's mastering a new command, overcoming a behavioural challenge, or simply sharing moments of joy, each step forward is a testament to your dedication and the resilience of your French Bulldog.

1. **Reflect on Achievements:** Consider the achievements and growth you and your Frenchie have experienced together. From the early days of puppyhood to the well-trained and well-adjusted dog before you, recognize the effort and commitment invested in this journey.

2. **Capture Memories:** Cherish the memories created throughout the training process. Document your Frenchie's antics, victories, and the special moments that have defined your shared experience. Photos, videos, and a journal can be wonderful ways to preserve these precious memories.

3. **Appreciate the Bond:** Take a moment to appreciate the deep bond forged between you and your French Bulldog. The mutual trust, companionship, and understanding are the

foundations of a lifelong connection that goes beyond training sessions.

4. Express Gratitude: Express gratitude for the joy and unconditional love your Frenchie brings into your life. Recognize the positive impact they have had on your well-being and the fulfilment they bring to your daily routines.

Continuous Learning and Adaptation

The journey of training and caring for a French Bulldog is an ongoing process that requires continuous learning and adaptation. As your Frenchie grows and evolves, so too must your approach to their well-being. Embrace the spirit of lifelong learning, understanding that each stage of your dog's life brings new opportunities and challenges.

1. Stay Informed: Stay abreast of the latest developments in dog care, training techniques, and veterinary practices. Regularly consult with your veterinarian and seek reputable sources for updated information on French Bulldog health and well-being.

2. Adapt to Changing Needs: Recognize that your Frenchie's needs will change over time. Whether it's adjusting their diet, modifying exercise routines, or adapting training methods, be flexible and responsive to their evolving requirements.

3. Continue Mental Stimulation: Dogs, especially intelligent breeds like the French Bulldog, thrive on mental stimulation. Introduce new toys, games, and training challenges to keep their minds sharp and engaged

4. Prioritize Health: Prioritize your Frenchie's health through regular vet checkups, preventive care, and a well-balanced diet. As they age, be vigilant for signs of common health issues and address them promptly.

5. Deepen the Bond: The bond between you and your French Bulldog is a dynamic and evolving connection. Invest time in activities that strengthen this bond, such as playtime, training sessions, and shared adventures.

In conclusion, the journey with your French Bulldog is not a destination but a continuous exploration filled with growth, joy, and mutual understanding. By celebrating achievements, expressing gratitude, and maintaining a commitment to continuous learning, you ensure that your Frenchie's life is enriched, and your relationship remains a source of joy and fulfillment for years to come.

Appendix

Additional Resources

1. Books:
  - "The French Bulldog Handbook" by Linda Whitwam
  - "French Bulldogs: Everything About Purchase, Care, Nutrition, Behaviour, and Training" by D. Caroline Coile, Ph.D.

2. Websites:
  - American Kennel Club (AKC) - https://www.akc.org/
  - French Bulldog Club of America (FBDCA) - https://frenchbulldogclub.org/
  - The French Bulldog Village - https://frenchbulldogvillage.net/

3. Online Communities:
  - French Bulldog Reddit Community - https://www.reddit.com/r/frogdogs/
  - French Bulldog Forum - https://www.frenchbulldognews.com/forum/

4. Training Apps:
   - Puppr - Dog Training & Tricks
   - Dogo - Your Dog's Favourite Training App

Training Logs and Charts

1. Training Session Log:
   - Date
   - Duration of the session
   - Training goals and objectives
   - Commands practiced
   - Notable observations or challenges

2. Behavioural Journal:
   - Date and time of observed behaviour
   - Description of the behaviour
   - Context or trigger of the behaviour
   - Your response or intervention
   - Outcome or resolution

3. Feeding and Exercise Schedule:
   - Daily feeding times and portion sizes
   - Duration and type of exercise
   - Notes on any changes in appetite or energy levels

Glossary of Terms

1. **Positive Reinforcement:** A training method that involves rewarding desired behaviours to encourage their repetition.

2. **Clicker Training:** A training technique that uses a clicker to provide immediate and precise feedback to a dog during training.

3. **Socialization:** The process of exposing a dog to various people, places, and situations to ensure they are well-adjusted and comfortable in different environments.

4. **Separation Anxiety:** A behavioural issue where a dog experiences distress when left alone, leading to behaviours like excessive barking, destructive chewing, or house soiling.

5. **No-Pull Harness:** A type of harness designed to discourage pulling by redirecting a dog's attention without causing discomfort.

6. **Counter-Conditioning:** A training technique that involves changing an animal's response to a specific stimulus by pairing it with a positive experience.

7. **Hypoallergenic:** Refers to foods or products designed to minimize the risk of triggering allergies.

8. **Glucosamine:** A supplement commonly used to support joint health, often given to senior dogs or those with arthritis.

9. **Cognitive Dysfunction:** A condition in senior dogs similar to dementia in humans, characterized by cognitive decline and changes in behaviour.

10. Joint Supplement: A supplement containing ingredients like glucosamine and chondroitin to support joint health, often used in senior dogs or those with arthritis.

This glossary provides a reference for key terms used throughout the book, and the training logs and charts in the appendix offer practical tools for tracking your French Bulldog's progress and maintaining organized training and care records.